NATURAL REMEDIES GUIDE FOR BEGINNERS

Natural Treatments and Herbal Recipes for Healing Yourself without Prescriptions and Achieving Fabulous, Skin and Body

ELIZABETH PARKER

Table of Contents

Introduction

I want to thank you and congratulate you for purchasing this book!

This book contains information as well as recipes that should help you not just understand the benefits of choosing natural products but also provide you with the knowledge you need to actually get started.

While you can easily buy natural products from different shops, it is often that they are priced much higher than the average. You might find yourself skipping them in order to save a few dollars on your purchase. However, that also means using stuff that might be damaging to your own health and body.

In this book, you'll be provided with easy to follow recipes which you can try at home without much hassle. The ingredients are easy to find and affordable so you can make homemade remedies without having to spend so much money. You can even give them out as gifts or sell them to friends.

Thanks again for purchasing this book, I hope you enjoy it! Please take some time to stop by and LIKE our Facebook page:

https://www.facebook.com/joypublishing

With gratitude,

ELIZABETH PARKER

Chapter 1

An Overview of Natural Treatments

When it comes to natural treatments or anything related to, among the first questions that you'll be asked would be: "Does it actually work?" Understandable, of course; as a great majority of us were raised to believe that if we're sick, the only remedy would be a prescription or over the counter drug. It has worked for us all our lives so why change it now? There are plenty of reasons why but we'll get to that a little later.

It is easy for people to dismiss herbal/plant-based remedies as no more than quackery. However what they forget is that long before the use of man-made medications, ancient healers and doctors have always turned to using botanicals when it came to their practice. There is a lot of literature on this; information that's been collected by the ancient doctors themselves and further developed in this day and age. In fact, some of these herbs? They serve as active ingredients for the medicines that you take today.

Before we get more in depth, let's talk about the advantages as well as the disadvantages that come with using natural treatments on yourself. This should allow you to better understand what you're getting into, especially if this is your first time trying it out.

Advantages

1. Reduced Side Effects Risk - Many herbal remedies are tolerated well by our bodies and when it comes to side effects, the cases of this is a lot lower when compared to the average pharmaceutical drug. Another thing worth mentioning is that in the long run, herbs are also less damaging to our bodies and internal organs. Do remember that constant use of certain medications can eventually wear your organs down-- the liver being the most at risk.

2. Effective for Chronic Conditions - For many people who have long standing health issues which no longer respond well to the medications being provided (due to various reasons; the most common of which is tolerance), the used of herbal medicines provide them with an effective alternative. One that's also more efficient when it comes to handling the symptoms without causing random flare outs and the like. For example, a medication called Vioxx, a relatively well-known prescription drug used for treating arthritis, was recalled after a number of people experienced an increase in their risk of cardiovascular complications.

This is where natural treatments enter the picture. Treatments for arthritis in the herbal world include small dietary changes. Adding herbs and taking out certain food items that can trigger the symptoms is among them. Simple yet effective.

3. Affordability - Of course, among the many concerns that people have when it comes to purchasing pharmaceuticals would be the price. For being a necessity that's essential to all of us, medicines don't come cheap and this introduces a whole new set of problems for people who can't really afford them. Luckily, they now have a choice. Herbs cost much less than your average prescription medicine and they are also relatively widespread. Some, you can choose to plant in your garden or in small-scale ones right in your kitchen. Not only is this convenient, but it also allows you to save your money and use it for something else. There are a lot of healing herbs and plants that you can grow right in the comfort of your own home-- regardless of the available space.

Disadvantages

Of course, herbs are not without disadvantages and there are times when they won't be appropriate to use. Here are some that you should consider.

4. Appropriateness - We have to admit that there are, in fact, certain illnesses that can be treated by modern medicine more effectively and efficiently. Among them, physical trauma such as a broken leg. Herbs will not be able to heal your appendicitis or a heart attack. For these things, modern medicine still remains to be the best option for you.

5. Side Effects Caused by Medication Interactions - Yes, there are certain cases wherein herbal remedies cause problems when used in conjunction with your prescriptions. Not all herbal remedies come with a warning and there are those, such as the Valerian, which can actually cause a chemical reaction when taken alongside other antidepressants. This is where open discussion with your physician comes in handy. Your doctor has to know if you plan on taking herbal remedies so that he or she can look into the possible effects that may come from it.

Can herbal medicine become a part of your regular treatment?

The answer would be yes for as long as you understand both risks and benefits that may come from it. It is still important to visit your physician and not just your herbalist to get a clearer picture of what you need to do and the things that you should avoid in order to prevent complications from happening.

Chapter 2

All Natural Treatments from your Cupboard

Turmeric: Having a helping of this could actually relieve the symptoms brought on by arthritis. This is because turmeric actually contains *curcumin*, a potent and natural anti-inflammatory that works in the same manner as Cox-2 inhibitors. It helps in reducing the Cox-2 enzyme which is the cause of swelling and pain when it comes to arthritis.

There are also studies that look into its effects when it comes to preventing both Alzheimer's disease and colon cancer. A clinical trial done by the John Hopkin's University showed that curcumin is capable of shrinking precancerous lesions (colon polyps) when taken together with a small amount of quercetin-- another powerful antioxidant which is found in apples, onions and cabbages.

Cinnamon: Despite the fact that it is a typical accompaniment of desserts such as ice cream, cinnamon can actually help in lowering your blood sugar. Besides that, there are studies being conducted to try and discover how it can help lower cholesterol levels in the body as well. For people who have type 2 diabetes, this is certainly great news as they can tackle 2 of the issues that they deal with by simply adding cinnamon to their everyday diet.

For this to have any effect, however, one needs to take 1gram capsules of cinnamon extract on a daily basis. Remember that even natural remedies do come with a dosage limit so make sure you don't go beyond the recommended amount.

Rosemary: Are you the kind of person who enjoys broiled, fried and grilled food a lot? Well, here's something you should know-- if you weren't aware of it yet-- meat that's been cooked at high temperatures actually create what's referred to as HCA's and are pretty potent carcinogens often implicated in different cancer types. However, HCA levels are reduced significantly whenever rosemary extract (a common herbal powder used in cooking) is mixed into the meat itself before it's cooked.

It also helps prevent carcinogens from binding with our DNA which is, as researchers have said, the first step in tumor formation. The studies that they have conducted all show that rosemary can help reduce the risks for both tumor formation and DNA damage. More research needs to be done at this point but experts say that rosemary has incredible potential for this purpose.

Ginger: Ginger can help you avoid stomach upset which can be caused by a number of different reasons; motion sickness, pregnancy and chemotherapy are just three of the common examples where it might come in handy. Among the different folk remedies, ginger is known to be the most effective. A potent antioxidant by itself, it works by blocking serotonin and its effects. This is a chemical which is produced by both our stomach and brain whenever we feel nausea. Ginger also hinders the production free radicals which is another common reason why we experience an upset stomach.

Aside from this, ginger is also known to be capable of reducing arthritis pain, lower blood pressure and decrease cancer risks. There are components in ginger that help in regulating our blood flow which then helps lower high blood pressure. It also comes with, anti-inflammatory properties which can help in easing the symptoms of arthritis. The same properties are also thought to kill ovarian cells better and much less "traumatizing" than chemotherapy. Of course, studies are still being done to find out just how effective it can be against cancer cells but the preliminary tests have been positive.

Holy Basil: Feeling stressed lately? This herb would help put you back in a serene place-- quite befitting of its name. It is a variety of the same basil plant you commonly use in pesto sauces but quite unlike it, holy basil is known to be effective at combating stress by increasing both adrenaline and noradrenaline levels in your body while decreasing serotonin at the same time. In fact, tea infused with it can help relieve both headaches and indigestion. Certainly better than popping a pill or two just to feel better.

Another thing that researchers are looking into is its effects on breast cancer. In clinical tests, tea made from holy basil was able to shrink tumors, decreased the blood supply to it and eventually stopped it from spreading further.

Garlic: Aside from the fact that garlic is very beneficial when it comes to maintaining cardiovascular healthy, it is also known to help in lowering cancer risks; colorectal and ovarian to be specific. A clinical test showed that after a year of taking garlic supplements as well as garlic extract, patients that had histories of colon polyps experienced not just a reduction in its size but saw a decrease in pre-cancerous growths as well. Going back to the beginning, garlic contains 70 different phytochemicals which, studies have shown, can effectively decrease blood pressure by at least 30 points. It can also help you avoid strokes by slowing down any arterial blockages.

Honey: Often used as a natural sweetener, honey also has valuable components that can be used for treating a number of different things-- not to mention the fact that it can also efficiently help in beautifying our skin. Honey is often used as a cure for asthma as well as the common cough. Sometimes, it is used as a treatment for hay fever. Besides these, it can be applied directly onto the skin as a treatment for healing sun burns, burns and even wounds. This is because of the fact that it hastens healing and because of its antibacterial properties, also helps in preventing infection. A quick trivia: Did you know that honey has been in use since 50 A.D.? Its healing ability is even mentioned in the Torah, Koran and the Bible.

Now that we've discussed a few of the most common natural remedies that you can easily find in your cupboard, let's move to how to use them and what else we can do to further improve their efficiency. After all, sometimes, a teaspoon of this and that isn't quite enough.

Chapter 3

Quick and Easy Recipes for Curing Common Ailments

FOR COUGHS, COLDS AND THE LIKE

Vitamin C Shot
(For winter and whenever you feel a cold coming on)

Ingredients:

- ½ a cup of boiling water
- 8 ounces of pitted dates
- 1 cup of cold water
- 1 cup of yogurt or milk
- 4 teaspoons of lemon juice
- 1 teaspoon of grated lemon peel
- 1 to 2 teaspoons of powdered vitamin C

Procedure:

1. Combine your dates and boiling water in a blender. Puree.

2. Stir in your other ingredients slowly and mix well.

3. After, freeze it until it becomes firm.

4. Once done, beat until it becomes smooth again then move to a square pan.

5. Cover it with plastic wrap and freeze it again until it becomes firm.

Black Pepper and Honey Tea
(For wet coughs and relieving its symptoms)

Ingredients:

- 1 teaspoon of freshly ground black pepper
- 2 tablespoons of honey
- Hot water

Procedure:

1. Mix all of your ingredients together, making sure everything is incorporated well. You wouldn't want to end up swallowing small bits of pepper while drinking.

2. Cover and let it steep for at least 15 minutes before straining out the undissolved bits.

3. Sip whenever needed.

Marshmallow Root
(Throat soreness and itchiness)

Ingredients:

- 2 tablespoons of marshmallow root
- 2 tablespoons of honey
- Hot water

Procedure:

1. Boil the marshmallow root for a few minutes to infuse it into your water.

2. Strain it before transferring to a mug.

3. Stir in your honey and mix well.

4. Drink warm to relieve sore throat and itchiness.

Amish Cough Syrup
(1 teaspoon a day for children, 1 tablespoon a day for adults)

Ingredients:

- Castor Oil
- Lemon Juice
- Honey

Procedure:

1. Mix the ingredients together in equal parts.

2. Make sure everything is combined properly before storing.

Nighttime Cold Remedy
(Works a bit like Nyquil and would allow you to sleep well at night)

Ingredients:

- ¼ cup of maple syrup
- 1 lemon
- ¼ cup of hot water
- 2 tablespoons of brandy

Procedure:

1. Squeeze the juice from your lemon.

2. Mix this juice with your maple syrup then add the hot water.

3. Add 2 tablespoons of brandy.

4. Drink before bed.

Elderberry Extract

(Effective for treating the flu. Take 2 tablespoons at a time)

Ingredients:

- ½ a cup of berries
- 8 cups of water
- ½ a cup of honey

Procedure:

1. Boil your berries in the water and allow it to simmer down into at least 2 cups of liquid. This should take about half an hour to 45 minutes.

2. Run it through a strainer then add your honey.

3. Mix well before refrigerating.

DIFFERENT SKIN PROBLEMS

Natural Anti-Fungal Treatment
(For rashes as well as athletes foot)

Ingredients:

- 2 tablespoons of boric acid
- 1 cup of cornstarch

Procedure:

1. Mix both powders together and transfer to a salt shaker.

2. Shake it well before using.

Honey and Oats for Sunburn
(Sunburn relief as well healing the skin)

Ingredients:

- Honey
- Uncooked oats
- Milk (optional)

Procedure:

1. Clean your skin very gently.

2. Using a cotton ball, dab some milk onto the sun burnt spot.

3. Apply the honey directly onto the affected area. Massage it slowly.

4. Pat the oats on top of it. You can do this to your face as well, using it as a mask.

5. Leave it on for at least 5 minutes before rinsing off with warm water.

Peppermint and Basil Leaves
(Relieving bug bites and itchiness)

Ingredients:

- Fresh peppermint leaves
- Fresh basil leaves

Procedure:

1. In a separate bowl, crush both leaves.

2. Leave these in the fridge for at least 15 minutes. This would make them even more cooling and soothing when applied to the skin.

3. Apply it generally to the areas where the itchiness. Don't mix the leaves together.

TOOTHACHE RELIEF

Clove and Peppermint Oil for Toothaches

Ingredients:

- A tablespoon of clove oil
- A tablespoon of peppermint oil

Procedure:

1. Wash your hands thoroughly or get some cotton swab.

2. Take some of the oil you prefer and directly apply this to the infected area.

3. Make sure you do this lightly and with as little pressure as you can.

4. You can also rub some of it onto your gums.

Saltwater Gargle

(For those not keen on using oils)

Ingredients:

- 1 tablespoon of rock salt
- 1 glass of lukewarm water

Procedure:

1. Dissolve the salt in the warm water.

2. Gargle with it until you feel the pain in your tooth slowly fade.

3. Rinse by gargling plain water after.

Apple Cider Vinegar Gargle
(Helps reduce swelling and pain)

Ingredients:

- 1 tablespoon of Apple Cider Vinegar
- 1 glass of water for rinsing

Procedure:

1. Simply keep the Apple cider vinegar in your mouth for a few minutes before spitting it out.

2. Do not swallow it and you may repeat it as much as you need to.

FOR REDUCING FEVER

Amish Lung Fever Salve
(Can be used as a warming rub for both colds and pneumonia)

Ingredients:

- 2 oz camphor
- 12 oz unsalted lard
- 3 oz beeswax
- 3 ox powdered rosin

Procedure:

1. Mix all of the above using a double boiler.

2. Once incorporated well, take it off the heat.

3. Add 2 tablespoons of raw linseed oil and 20ml of turpentine.

4. Keep it in a sanitized bottle.

Egg White Socks

(This is meant to draw the heat from your head down to your feet.)

Ingredients:

- 2 to 3 organic egg whites for children and 5 for adults
- A clean pair of socks or a pair of small towels

Procedure:

1. Separate the yolk from your egg whites.

2. Soak your socks or towel in it for at least 15 minutes.

3. Put it on your feet or, if you're using a towel, wrap it snugly around each foot.

4. Leave this on for at least half an hour.

Garlic Foot Paste
(Anti-viral and helps with fighting off the infection)

Ingredients:

- Mashed garlic
- Olive or coconut oil

Procedure:

1. Mix the 2 ingredients together, making sure garlic turns into a paste-like consistency. You can use a processor for this if you have one.

2. Make sure it's not watery.

3. Spread it over the patient's foot, leaving spaces where heat can escape.

4. Wrap it in gauze and leave overnight.

*Note: This might seem a little too much for some considering the fact that garlic has a strong smell. Younger children might have trouble with it more than adults would. Try the alternative recipe below if you're not keen with this one.

Garlic Tablets
(Antiviral, antibacterial and will help fight off infection)

Ingredients:

- Natural garlic powder
- Fresh garlic, sliced into small pieces
- Honey
- Warm water

Procedure:

You have 2 options.

1. The first one is to eat the garlic fresh, sliced and peeled. The taste can be a little too strong for some so taking a teaspoon of honey would help with that.

2. The second option is to take some garlic powder and empty capsules. You'll fill these capsules with the powder and take it the same way you would a pill. This prevents you from actually tasting the garlic.

DIGESTIVE AND STOMACH PROBLEMS

Quick Cure for a Sour Stomach
(Acidity and Heartburn)

Ingredients:

- ½ a glass of water
- ½ a teaspoon of baking soda

Procedure:

1. Mix the two together, making sure it gets incorporated well.

2. Take this drink every two hours until the pain subsides.

3. The max would be 8 half teaspoons for adults that are below the age of 60 and 4 half-teaspoons for those who are over 60.

Castor Oil Constipation Relief

(Proven effective when it comes to adult constipation)

Ingredients:

- 1 tablespoon of castor oil
- A glass of warm milk or a cup of tea

Procedure:

1. Add a tablespoon of the castor oil into your warm milk or tea.

2. Mix this well and drink before bed.

3. You can also add half a teaspoon of honey if the taste is something you're not very fond of.

Warm Lemon Water

(Helps with indigestion, acidity and inflammation)

Ingredients:

- 1 fresh lemon
- Warm water
- Honey

Procedure:

1. Juice your lemon thoroughly and strain the seeds out.

2. Mix this with some water and add a smidge of honey.

Chapter 4

All Natural Beauty Solutions for the Hair and Skin

HAIR CARE

pH Balanced Natural Shampoo

Ingredients:

- ¾ cups of pure aloe vera gel
- 1 can of natural coconut milk
- Your favorite essential oil

Procedure:

1. Mix all of your ingredients together in a clean bowl. Make sure everything is incorporated properly.

2. Pour this mixture into ice cube trays. You might need 2.

3. Place it in the freezer until it becomes frozen completely.

4. To use it, simply take a cube out (or however many you need) the night before and keep it in a small contain in your fridge until you have to use it.

5. Use as you would your normal shampoo. Note that it will not lather.

Banana and Coconut Hair Conditioner

Ingredients:

- 1 banana
- 1 egg
- 1 tablespoon of coconut oil
- 1 tablespoon of honey

Procedure:

1. Mash your banana and mix it with the egg. Mix well.

2. Add a tablespoon of coconut oil to the mix

3. Add your honey and blend well.

4. Apply it generously and thoroughly all over your hair.

5. Leave it on for 30 minutes before rinsing it off with warm water and shampoo.

Coconut Oil Hair Moisturizer

Ingredients:

- ¾ cups of melted virgin coconut oil
- 1 tablespoon of honey
- 1/8 teaspoon of vitamin E oil
- 10 drops of your preferred essential oil

Procedure:

Mix your essential oil, vitamin E, honey and coconut oil (melted).

Once done, apply it to the ends of your hair while slowly working your way up. Make sure it's applied evenly.

Comb it through the strands of your hair using a wide tooth comb.

Wrap your hair in a shower cap.

Leave it on for an hour or two before rinsing it off.

FACIAL TREATMENTS

All Natural Acne Solution

Ingredients:

- 2 tablespoons of coconut oil
- 3 to 4 drops of purification oil

Tools:

- Eye dropper
- Lipbalm tubes

Procedure:

1. Using a small pot, melt your coconut oil. Once done, take it off the heat and stir in your purification oil.

2. Make sure everything is incorporated well before taking your eye dropper and using it to transfer the mixture to your lip balm tubes.

3. Place it in the fridge for a few hours until it hardens again.

4. Dab on areas where you have zits. It will dry it up and heal the broken skin as well.

Homemade Vitamin C Facial Serum

Ingredients:

- 1 teaspoon of vitamin c powder
- 1 teaspoon of glycerin
- 1 teaspoon of distilled water
- 1/8 teaspoon of vitamin e

Procedure:

1. Mix all of your ingredients until the granules in it are dissolved.

2. Transfer it to a dark glass bottle.

3. Apply during the evenings, after you're done with cleansing and toning.

Sun-kissed Glow Moisturizing Oil

Ingredients:

- 2 tablespoons of grape seed oil
- 1 tablespoon of hazelnut oil
- 1 tablespoon of borage seed oil
- 1 tablespoon of hemp seed oil

Procedure:

1. Mix all of your ingredients together.

2. Transfer it to a dark colored glass bottle and keep in a cool but dry place.

Seaweed Hydrating Face Mask

Ingredients:

- 1 teaspoon of honey
- 1 teaspoon of bladder wrack powder
- ¼ teaspoon of water

Procedure:

1. Mix your seaweed and honey in a clean dish. Add water to thin it out to the consistency you want to. ¼ teaspoon of water should be good enough.

2. Apply it evenly onto your face and allow to dry for about 20 minutes.

3. Rinse it off with warm water.

BODY ESSENTIALS

Safflower Silky Body Cream

Ingredients:

- 1 cup of shea butter
- ½ cup of safflower oil
- ½ cup of coconut oil
- 20 drops of essential oil

Procedure:

1. Using a double boiler, slowly melt your shea butter. Once melted completely, remove it from the heat and transfer this to a mixing bowl.

2. Stir in your add safflower and mix properly.

3. Place your bowl in your freezer until it begins to firm up again. This could take half an hour to 2 hours depending on your fridge.

4. Once it firms up, remove it from the cold and add your essential oils.

5. Using a whisk or a stand mixer, begin to whip it until you get the consistency that you want. This should take no more than 5 minutes at most.

6. Scoop your cream into a sanitized jar and store in a cool place.

Mineral Salt Deodorant Body Spray

Ingredients:

- Organic Witch Hazel
- Any essential oil of your choice
- Baking Soda
- Himalayan Salt
- Grapefruit Seed Extract

Procedure:

1. Measure out ¼ teaspoon of baking soda and 2 tablespoons of Himalayan salt. Put these into a clean bowl.

2. Add 5 tablespoons of organic witch hazel

3. Mix everything together until every granule of the baking soda has been dissolved.

4. Allow it to settle and pass it through a strainer.

5. Transfer to your spray bottle then add about 20 drops of your favorite essential oil.

6. Add 2 drops of grapefruit seed extract.

7. Shake well before using.

Beach Body Polish
(Gentle but effective exfoliant)

Ingredients:

- ½ a cup of coconut oil
- ¼ cup of Epsom salt
- ¼ cup of finely ground sea salt
- 2 teaspoons of concentrated liquid minerals
- 10 drops of your preferred essential oil (optional)

Procedure:

1. Put your coconut oil in a bowl. If it's a little stiff, mash it continuously until it becomes soft enough for you to mix properly.

2. Add your Epsom and sea salt. Stir this until it gets blended evenly.

3. Add your liquid minerals as well as your essential oils if you're using any. Stir it again until everything is well incorporated.

4. You can use this body scrub for exfoliating twice a week depending on the need.

Homemade Sea Salt Bath

(Relieves aches and pains as well as exfoliates)

Ingredients:

- 1 cup of sea salt
- 1 cup of Epsom salts
- 2 tablespoons of concentrated sea minerals
- ¼ teaspoon of vitamin c crystals

Procedure:

1. Simply add all of your ingredients into your tub once it's been filled with water.

2. Make sure the water is warm so it adds another relaxing factor to it.

3. Soak for at least half an hour before rinsing off.

Antioxidant Coffee Body Scrub

Ingredients:

- 1 cup of organic coffee (grounded)
- 1 cup of organic sugar (or salt)
- ½ a cup of organic coconut oil
- ½ tablespoon of vanilla
- ½ tablespoon of cinnamon

Procedure:

1. Melt your coconut oil, allowing it to cool after but don't let it solidify again.

2. Once it's cooled down, add your other ingredients to it and mix well.

3. Store in an air-tight container and use whenever needed.

Chapter 5

All Natural Health and Skin Care Recipes for Kids

Kid-friendly Detoxifying Bath

Ingredients:

- Epsom salt or magnesium flakes
- Coconut or olive oil
- Your preferred essential oil
- Baking soda if your water is unfiltered
- Warm tub of water

Procedure:

1. Add your Epsom salt/magnesium flakes to the water. 2 cups would be the max for adults while for younger children, it would be 1 cup.

2. Add your baking soda if needed. A cup is the max.

3. Add your coconut oil/olive oil. 3 tablespoons is the max for adults and 2 tablespoons for children.

4. Add your essential oils. 10 drops is the max for adults while 6 drops is the max for children.

5. Only use it on their bodies as getting this mixture in the hair can make it very greasy due to the coconut oil.

6. Let them soak for half an hour or much less before rinsing off.

All Natural Diaper Rash Treatment Stick

Ingredients:

- 3 tablespoons of grated beeswax
- 2 tablespoons of coconut oil
- 1 tablespoon of shea butter
- 1 tablespoon of jojoba oil
- 10 drops of your favorite essential oil

Procedure:

1. Using a double boiler over low heat, melt your beeswax.

2. Once it's melted, add your jojoba oil, coconut oil and shea butter. Wait for everything to melt and mix together. Stir it gently.

3. Remove this from the heat and allow it to cool down a bit before adding your essential oils. Use very little if it's scented especially if your baby is under 6 months of age.

4. Once it's cooled bit, pour it into a used deodorant container. Make sure it's been sanitized and cleaned.

5. Keep it in the fridge so it solidifies quickly.

Conclusion

Thank you again for purchasing this book!

I hope this book was able to help you to better understand the benefits of going all natural when it comes to treating certain ailments as well as beautifying your hair and skin.

The next step is to take the things that you have learned and give them a try. From the recipes to simply learning more about the best natural cures available for you. This is knowledge that you'll certainly benefit a lot from and not just on a personal care level. Many people have used this knowledge, expanded on it and created small businesses that teach as well as provide other like-minded people with an opportunity to try it for themselves.

In addition, please remember to check out our Facebook page in order to find other resources and upcoming promotions:

https://www.facebook.com/joypublishing

With sincere thanks,

ELIZABETH PARKER

One Last Thing...

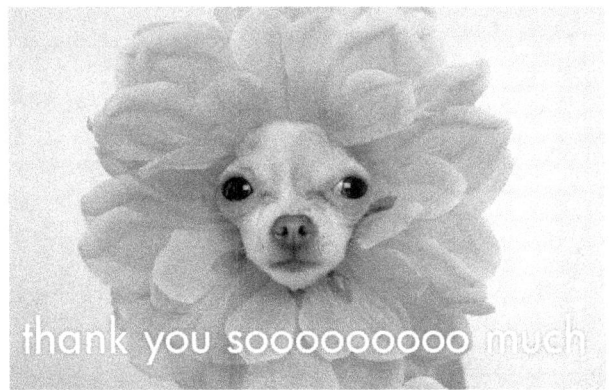

Source: Wikipedia

If you believe that this book is worth sharing, would you please take the time to let others know how it affected your life? If it turns out to make a difference in the lives of others, they will be forever grateful to you, as will I.

www.ingramcontent.com/pod-product-compliance
Lightning Source LLC
Chambersburg PA
CBHW060650290526
45793CB00001B/472